# The Rhythm Within

## Understanding Blood Pressure

By

Walter B. Scoville

Vol one

## Disclaimer

The information contained in this book is for general informational purposes only. The author and publisher have made every effort to ensure the accuracy and completeness of the content within this book, but make no representations or warranties of any kind, express or implied, about the completeness, accuracy, reliability, suitability, or availability with respect to the book or the information, products, services, or related graphics contained in the book for any purpose.

The content of this book is not intended to be a substitute for professional advice, diagnosis, or treatment. Always seek the advice of a qualified professional with any questions you may have regarding a particular topic. The author and publisher disclaim any liability for any actions taken or not taken based on the information provided in this book.

The views and opinions expressed in this book are solely those of the author and do not necessarily reflect the official policy or position of any organization, institution, or individual mentioned within. Any resemblance to actual events, locales, or persons, living or dead, is purely coincidental.

The author and publisher have exerted their best efforts in preparing this book, but make no representations or warranties with respect to the accuracy or completeness of the contents. They assume no liability for errors or omissions or for any damages resulting from the use of the information contained in this book.

All trademarks, service marks, trade names, and logos referenced in this book belong to their respective owners and are used for identification purposes only. The inclusion of such references does not imply any endorsement by the author or publisher.

Any unauthorized use or distribution of the content of this book is strictly prohibited. This includes but is not limited to copying, sharing, reproducing, or transmitting any part of the book in any form or by any means, electronic or mechanical, including photocopying, recording, or any information storage and retrieval system, without prior written permission from the author and publisher.

Every effort has been made to accurately credit and acknowledge all sources used in this book. If any omission or error has occurred, it is unintentional, and the author and publisher will be pleased to rectify it in future editions or reprints.

By reading this book, you acknowledge and agree to the terms and conditions stated in this disclaimer

Table Of Content

# **INTRODUCTION**

"The Rhythm Within: Understanding Blood Pressure" is a comprehensive guide that takes you on a journey through the intricate workings of blood pressure and its significance for your overall health. In this book, we will delve deep into the complexities of blood pressure, unraveling its mysteries, and equipping you with the knowledge necessary to take control of your cardiovascular well-being.

In today's fast-paced world, where stress, sedentary lifestyles, and poor dietary choices have become the norm, maintaining optimal blood pressure levels has become increasingly crucial. Through this book, we aim to provide you with a holistic understanding of blood pressure, including its measurement, factors that influence it, associated health conditions, and effective management strategies.

Each chapter of "The Rhythm Within: Understanding Blood Pressure" focuses on a specific aspect related to blood pressure. From deciphering the terminology to exploring the various diagnostic tools and techniques used, you will gain a comprehensive understanding of how blood pressure is measured and interpreted. Additionally, we will shed light on the dangers of high blood pressure, commonly known as hypertension, and discuss the medications available for its control.

Furthermore, we will examine the lifestyle factors that significantly impact blood pressure, such as diet, exercise, stress, and age. You will discover practical tips and evidence-based strategies to adopt healthier habits that promote optimal blood pressure levels. We will also address the unique considerations surrounding blood pressure during pregnancy and childhood, offering guidance to both expectant mothers and parents.

"The Rhythm Within: Understanding Blood Pressure" goes beyond conventional approaches to blood pressure management. We will explore alternative and complementary therapies, encouraging a holistic approach to enhance your overall well-being. By integrating mind, body, and spirit, you can unlock the power to regulate your blood pressure and lead a healthier, more fulfilling life.

# CHAPTER ONE

# Introduction To Blood Pressure

Blood pressure is a fundamental physiological measurement that provides crucial insights into the cardiovascular health of an individual. It is often referred to as the "silent killer" because high blood pressure, also known as hypertension, can go unnoticed for extended periods while causing significant damage to the body. In this chapter, we will explore the importance of understanding blood pressure and its impact on overall well-being.

Blood pressure is a reflection of the force exerted by circulating blood against the walls of the arteries. It is measured in millimeters of mercury (mmHg) and consists of two values: systolic pressure and diastolic pressure. Systolic pressure represents the pressure exerted on the arterial walls when the heart contracts and pumps blood into the circulation. Diastolic pressure, on the other hand, signifies the pressure in the arteries when the heart is at rest between contractions.

Monitoring blood pressure is a vital aspect of routine medical check-ups and plays a crucial role in identifying potential health risks. By understanding the principles behind blood pressure measurement, individuals can take proactive steps to manage and maintain healthy blood pressure levels, thereby reducing the risk of cardiovascular diseases.

The measurement of blood pressure is typically performed using a device called a sphygmomanometer. This device consists of an inflatable cuff that is wrapped around the upper arm, a pressure gauge to measure the pressure, and a stethoscope to detect the sounds of blood flow. The cuff is inflated to a level that temporarily restricts blood flow in the brachial artery. As the pressure in the cuff is gradually released, the healthcare professional listens for specific sounds known as Korotkoff sounds using the stethoscope. These sounds indicate the return of blood flow as the cuff pressure decreases, allowing the determination of systolic and diastolic pressure values.

Blood pressure readings are expressed as a fraction, with the systolic pressure appearing as the numerator and the diastolic pressure as the denominator. For instance, a reading of 120/80 mmHg indicates a systolic pressure of 120 mmHg and a diastolic pressure of 80 mmHg. It is essential to understand these numbers and their significance in assessing overall cardiovascular health.

Maintaining healthy blood pressure levels is crucial as persistent high blood pressure can lead to serious complications, including heart disease, stroke, kidney problems, and damage to blood vessels. Regular blood pressure monitoring allows individuals to track changes over time and identify any deviations from the optimal range. This information enables healthcare providers to implement appropriate interventions such as lifestyle modifications, medications, and other treatment strategies to manage blood pressure effectively.

# CHAPTER TWO

# How Blood Pressure Is Measured

Accurate measurement of blood pressure is essential for assessing cardiovascular health and identifying potential risks associated with hypertension. In this chapter, we will delve into the process of measuring blood pressure, the equipment used, and the techniques employed to obtain reliable readings.

The most common method used to measure blood pressure is through the use of a sphygmomanometer, a device that consists of an inflatable cuff, a pressure gauge, and a stethoscope. This instrument enables healthcare professionals to obtain precise readings by assessing the blood flow through the brachial artery.

The blood pressure measurement process typically involves the following steps:

**Preparation:** The individual should be in a relaxed state, sitting or lying down comfortably. It is recommended to avoid consuming caffeinated beverages, smoking, or engaging in vigorous physical activity immediately before the measurement, as these factors can temporarily elevate blood pressure.
**Positioning:** The individual's arm should be positioned at heart level,

supported by a surface such as a table or armrest. This positioning minimizes the effect of gravity on blood pressure measurements.

**Cuff Placement:** The cuff of the sphygmomanometer is wrapped around the upper arm, just above the elbow. It should be snug but not excessively tight. The healthcare professional ensures that the cuff is properly positioned and aligned with the brachial artery.

**Inflation:** The cuff is inflated by pumping air into it using a hand bulb or an automated mechanism. This inflation temporarily occludes blood flow in the brachial artery.

**Auscultation:** The healthcare professional listens for Korotkoff sounds using a stethoscope placed over the brachial artery. These sounds indicate the resumption of blood flow as the pressure in the cuff is gradually released.

**Deflation:** The cuff pressure is slowly released at a controlled rate. As the pressure decreases, the healthcare professional continues to listen for the Korotkoff sounds.

**Determining Systolic and Diastolic Pressure:** The systolic pressure is identified as the first sound heard, which corresponds to the point when blood flow becomes detectable. The diastolic pressure is determined as the point when the Korotkoff sounds disappear completely, indicating that blood flow has been fully restored. It is important to note that obtaining accurate blood pressure measurements requires proper technique and attentiveness to ensure reliable results. Factors such as cuff size, positioning, and the proficiency of the healthcare professional can impact the accuracy of readings. Regular calibration and maintenance of the sphygmomanometer are also necessary to ensure its proper functioning. In recent years, automated blood pressure monitors have become increasingly popular for home use. These devices utilize oscillometric technology to measure blood pressure and eliminate the need for a stethoscope. Automated monitors are user-friendly and provide convenient self-measurement options, although they may have certain limitations compared to manual measurements.

# CHAPTER THREE

## Understanding Blood Pressure Readings

Blood pressure readings provide valuable information about an individual's cardiovascular health. By understanding how to interpret these readings, we can gain insights into the condition of the cardiovascular system and assess the risk of potential health complications. In this chapter, we will explore the significance of systolic and diastolic pressure values and discuss the range of blood pressure readings.

Blood pressure readings are expressed as a fraction, with the systolic pressure as the numerator and the diastolic pressure as the denominator. For instance, a blood pressure reading of 120/80 mmHg indicates a systolic pressure of 120 mmHg and a diastolic pressure of 80 mmHg. Both values are essential in evaluating cardiovascular health.

**Systolic Pressure:** The systolic pressure represents the maximum force exerted on the arterial walls when the heart contracts and pumps blood into the circulation. It is an indicator of the pressure within the arteries during ventricular contraction. Systolic pressure is influenced by factors such as cardiac output, arterial compliance, and peripheral resistance. Normal systolic pressure typically ranges between 90 and 120 mmHg.

**Diastolic Pressure:** The diastolic pressure represents the pressure within the arteries when the heart is at rest between contractions. It reflects the minimum force exerted on the arterial walls during the relaxation phase of the cardiac cycle. Diastolic pressure is influenced by factors such as arterial tone, peripheral resistance, and vascular elasticity. Normal diastolic pressure typically ranges between 60 and 80 mmHg.

Interpreting blood pressure readings involves considering both systolic and diastolic pressures together. Here are the commonly recognized blood pressure categories:

**Normal Blood Pressure:** A normal blood pressure reading falls within the range of approximately 90/60 mmHg to 120/80 mmHg. This indicates that the cardiovascular system is functioning efficiently, and there is a balanced flow of blood through the arteries.

**Elevated Blood Pressure:** Elevated blood pressure is a category introduced by the American Heart Association (AHA) to identify individuals at higher risk of developing hypertension. Readings between 120/80 mmHg and 129/80 mmHg fall within this category. While not classified as hypertension, elevated blood pressure serves as a warning sign that lifestyle modifications may be necessary to prevent the progression of hypertension.

## Hypertension Stage 1:

Hypertension Stage 1 represents the initial stage of high blood pressure. It is characterized by systolic pressure ranging from 130 mmHg to 139 mmHg or diastolic pressure ranging from 80 mmHg to 89 mmHg. At this stage, healthcare professionals often recommend lifestyle changes, such as dietary modifications and increased physical activity, to manage blood pressure.

## Hypertension Stage 2:

Hypertension Stage 2 indicates more advanced high blood pressure. It involves systolic pressure of 140 mmHg or higher, or diastolic pressure of 90 mmHg or higher. At this stage, healthcare professionals may consider prescribing antihypertensive medications in addition to lifestyle modifications to control blood pressure.

**Hypertensive Crisis:**
A hypertensive crisis occurs when blood pressure reaches severely high levels, posing immediate health risks. Systolic pressure exceeding 180 mmHg and/or diastolic pressure exceeding 120 mmHg falls into this category. A hypertensive crisis requires prompt medical attention to prevent organ damage and other severe complications.

# CHAPTER FOUR

## Factors Affecting Blood Pressure

Blood pressure can be influenced by various factors, including age, genetics, lifestyle choices, underlying health conditions, and medications. Understanding these factors is crucial for comprehending the complexities of blood pressure regulation and its impact on overall cardiovascular health. In this chapter, we will explore the key factors that can affect blood pressure levels.

**Age:** Blood pressure tends to increase with age due to changes in arterial stiffness and decreased elasticity of blood vessels. As individuals get older, their blood vessels become less flexible, resulting in increased resistance to blood flow and higher blood pressure. This age-related increase in blood pressure highlights the importance of regular blood pressure monitoring, particularly among older adults.

**Genetics:** Genetic factors play a significant role in determining an individual's susceptibility to high blood pressure. Certain genetic variations can predispose individuals to hypertension by affecting the regulation of blood vessel constriction, sodium balance, and kidney function. Understanding the genetic components of blood pressure regulation can aid in identifying individuals at higher risk and implementing preventive measures.

**Lifestyle Choices:** Several lifestyle choices can significantly impact blood pressure levels. Unhealthy habits such as a diet high in sodium, saturated fats, and cholesterol can contribute to hypertension. Lack of physical activity, excessive alcohol consumption, and tobacco use are also associated with elevated blood pressure. Making positive lifestyle changes, such as adopting a balanced diet, engaging in regular exercise, limiting alcohol intake, and avoiding tobacco, can help maintain healthy blood pressure levels.

**Underlying Health Conditions:** Certain medical conditions can influence blood pressure. Chronic conditions such as kidney disease, diabetes, and hormonal disorders like Cushing's syndrome or hyperthyroidism can contribute to hypertension. Additionally, sleep apnea, a disorder characterized by interrupted breathing during sleep, is closely associated with high blood pressure. Proper management of these underlying health conditions is essential for controlling blood pressure.

**Medications:** Certain medications can affect blood pressure levels. Some medications, such as nonsteroidal anti-inflammatory drugs (NSAIDs), decongestants, and oral contraceptives, may lead to temporary increases in blood pressure. Conversely, antihypertensive medications are prescribed to lower blood pressure in individuals with hypertension. It is important for healthcare professionals to carefully consider the effects of medications on blood pressure and make appropriate adjustments when necessary.

**Stress:** Chronic stress can have a significant impact on blood pressure. When individuals experience stress, their body releases stress hormones like cortisol, which can temporarily raise blood pressure. Prolonged or frequent exposure to stress can contribute to sustained increases in blood pressure. Implementing stress management techniques such as relaxation exercises, mindfulness practices, and engaging in activities that promote emotional well-being can help reduce the impact of stress on blood pressure.

Understanding the various factors that influence blood pressure allows individuals to take proactive steps in maintaining healthy levels. By making informed lifestyle choices, managing underlying health conditions, and adhering to prescribed medications, individuals can effectively control their blood pressure and reduce the risk of associated complications. In the next chapter, we will explore the intricate mechanisms involved in the regulation of blood pressure within the body.

# CHAPTER FIVE

# Regulation Of Blood Pressure

Maintaining optimal blood pressure is a dynamic process regulated by a complex interplay of physiological mechanisms within the body. In this chapter, we will explore the intricate systems responsible for blood pressure regulation and understand how they work together to ensure the stability of cardiovascular health.

The Renin-Angiotensin-Aldosterone System (RAAS): The RAAS is a vital hormonal system involved in blood pressure regulation. When blood pressure drops or there is a decrease in blood volume, specialized cells in the kidneys release an enzyme called renin. Renin acts on a protein called angiotensinogen, which is produced in the liver, to form angiotensin I. Angiotensin I is then converted to angiotensin II by the action of an enzyme called angiotensin-converting enzyme (ACE). Angiotensin II causes vasoconstriction, narrowing the blood vessels and increasing blood pressure. It also stimulates the release of aldosterone, a hormone that promotes sodium and water retention by the kidneys, leading to an increase in blood volume.

**The Sympathetic Nervous System:** The sympathetic nervous system plays a crucial role in blood pressure regulation through its control over heart rate, blood vessel constriction, and cardiac output. When blood pressure drops, specialized receptors called baroreceptors located in the arteries detect the change and send signals to the brain. In response, the sympathetic nervous system is activated, leading to increased heart rate, stronger cardiac contractions, and vasoconstriction. These actions work collectively to raise blood pressure.

**The Endothelial System:** The endothelium, the inner lining of blood vessels, plays a pivotal role in blood pressure regulation. It releases various substances, including nitric oxide, prostacyclin, and endothelin, that influence blood vessel dilation and constriction. Nitric oxide, for example, causes blood vessels to relax and widen, promoting increased blood flow and decreased blood pressure. Imbalances in these endothelial factors can contribute to the development of hypertension.

**Kidney Function:** The kidneys play a critical role in long-term blood pressure regulation through their control over fluid balance and sodium excretion. When blood pressure is high, the kidneys filter and excrete excess sodium and water, reducing blood volume and subsequently lowering blood pressure. Conversely, when blood pressure is low, the kidneys conserve sodium and water, leading to increased blood volume and elevation of blood pressure.

**Other Factors:** Several additional factors influence blood pressure regulation. Hormones such as atrial natriuretic peptide (ANP) and brain natriuretic peptide (BNP) promote sodium and water excretion, helping to reduce blood volume and lower blood pressure. Additionally, factors like oxygen levels, carbon dioxide levels, and the viscosity of blood also affect blood pressure regulation.

Understanding the intricate mechanisms involved in blood pressure regulation highlights the importance of maintaining a delicate balance within the cardiovascular system. Disruptions in these regulatory systems can lead to the development of hypertension or hypotension, both of which can have adverse effects on overall health. By comprehending the complex interplay of these mechanisms, healthcare professionals can devise targeted strategies to manage blood pressure effectively.

In the next chapter, we will delve deeper into the risks associated with high blood pressure and the potential complications that can arise from uncontrolled hypertension.

# CHAPTER SIX

# Importance Of Monitoring Pressure

High blood pressure, also known as hypertension, is a significant health concern that affects millions of individuals worldwide. In this chapter, we will explore the risks associated with high blood pressure and the potential complications that can arise from uncontrolled hypertension.

Increased Risk of Cardiovascular Disease: High blood pressure is a leading risk factor for cardiovascular diseases such as heart attack, stroke, and heart failure. Persistent elevation in blood pressure can cause damage to the walls of arteries, leading to the formation of plaque and narrowing of the blood vessels. This condition, known as atherosclerosis, restricts blood flow to vital organs and increases the risk of cardiovascular events.

## Organ Damage:

Uncontrolled hypertension can result in damage to various organs in the body. The constant strain on blood vessels can lead to the weakening and enlargement of the heart, a condition called left ventricular hypertrophy. Over time, this can impair the heart's ability to pump blood effectively and may lead to heart failure. High blood pressure can also affect the kidneys, causing chronic kidney disease or even kidney failure.

Increased Risk of Stroke: Hypertension is a major risk factor for stroke, a condition characterized by the interruption of blood flow to the brain. High blood pressure can weaken the blood vessel walls, making them more susceptible to rupture or leakage. This can result in a hemorrhagic stroke, where bleeding occurs in the brain. Additionally, hypertension can lead to the formation of blood clots, increasing the risk of an ischemic stroke, which occurs when a clot blocks a blood vessel in the brain.

**Eye Complications:**
Chronic hypertension can damage the blood vessels in the eyes,

leading to various eye complications. Hypertensive retinopathy occurs when the tiny blood vessels in the retina become damaged and can result in vision problems or even vision loss. High blood pressure can also increase the risk of other eye conditions such as glaucoma and optic neuropathy.

**Aneurysm:**
High blood pressure can contribute to the formation of an aneurysm, which is a bulging or weakened area in the wall of an artery. The constant force of blood against the weakened artery can cause it to rupture, leading to severe internal bleeding and potentially life-threatening consequences.

**Metabolic Syndrome and Diabetes:** Hypertension is often associated with metabolic syndrome, a cluster of conditions that includes abdominal obesity, high blood sugar levels, high triglyceride levels, low HDL cholesterol levels, and insulin resistance. These factors increase the risk of developing type 2 diabetes, further exacerbating the complications associated with high blood pressure.

Cognitive Decline: Studies have suggested a link between high blood pressure and cognitive decline, including an increased risk of developing dementia and Alzheimer's disease. The exact mechanisms underlying this association are still being investigated, but it is believed that hypertension's impact on blood vessel health and blood flow to the brain may play a role.

Managing and controlling blood pressure through lifestyle modifications and appropriate medical interventions is crucial for reducing the risks and complications associated with hypertension. Regular blood pressure monitoring, adherence to prescribed medications, maintaining a healthy weight, adopting a balanced diet low in sodium, engaging in regular physical activity, managing stress, and avoiding tobacco and excessive alcohol consumption are all essential steps in maintaining optimal blood pressure levels and mitigating potential complications.

In the next chapter, we will explore the various lifestyle modifications and treatment options available for effectively managing high blood pressure.

47